Samara Gomes

Dental caries in adolescents in the city of Recife - PE

Samara Gomes

Dental caries in adolescents in the city of Recife - PE

Dental caries in adolescents in the city of Recife - PE, Brazil

ScienciaScripts

DEDICATORY

To God, for his strength and for never abandoning me during this long journey.

To *my parents, who, with great affection and support, spared no effort to get me to this stage of my life.*

To *my dear supervisor and professor Silvia Regina Sampaio, for her patience, affection and encouragement, which made it possible to complete this work.*

ACKNOWLEDGEMENTS

To **God**, the centre and foundation of everything in my life, for renewing my strength and disposition at every moment and for the discernment granted throughout this journey. I am grateful to him for the gift of life, for his infinite love.

To my dear supervisor, Professor **Silvia Regina Sampaio Bezerra**, who was with me from my first steps in the clinic to the end, thank you for your patience, affection, smiles and teachings. You were the one who believed in me, listened patiently to my considerations, shared your ideas, knowledge and experiences with me and always calmed me down by finding a solution to everything. I would like to express my recognition and admiration for your professional competence and my gratitude for your friendship, for being an extremely qualified professional. Thank you for your love, care, attention and dedication. I will miss you very much!

To my beloved mother, **Marineide**, who dedicated her life to my future, overcoming barriers and helping me to achieve victories. She who never let go of my hand in the face of life's difficulties and seeing my anguish always said at the end of everything the phrase "va/ *dar tudo certo*", My warrior mother, the mirror of my life, she who always prays for me and who believed that I would be able to achieve everything. Thank you for the sacrifices you made throughout my long journey, this achievement is also yours.

To my great father, **Livani**, for his advice, every encouragement and guidance, for his prayers in my favour, for his concern that I should always be walking the right path.

To my brother, **Hugo**, who accompanied me all the time I lived in Recife, from high school to college, for the nights teaching me physics for the entrance exam, for the encouragement that I could learn everything, for the advice, for the protection, for the companionship and friendship, I admire you a lot.

My aunts, **Marinalva and Maricélia**, my second mums, who helped me and hugged me all this time, always believing in me, thank you for your advice, help and concern.

To Professor **Ronaldo de Carvalho**, for his teachings and assistance in carrying out this research.

To Professor **Adriane Tenório**, one of the teachers who made me love endodontics, thank you for your teachings throughout this journey.

To my dear friend, **Thaís Albert**, who has been supporting me in my work and helping me edit this one. Thank you for your friendship, affection and patience in my absence.

To my classmates, especially my partner in the clinics at university, **Raíssa Arruda**, who was with me every day, teaching me, laughing and going through sorrows and joys, and who will be sharing another great victory. Thank you, because I was able to find in you a true sister and become more and more convinced of God's goodness, because having you as my partner during these years has been incredible! Thank you for all your affection, patience and the moments when we learnt so much together. You are a gift from God.

To my **fellow students**, who in some way have made my academic life more challenging every day. I ask God to bless you greatly, filling your paths with peace, love, health and prosperity.

I would like to thank **Vera Lúcia Pereira, a** dental surgeon with the PE Military Police, for her advice, teachings and research guidance. I will carry your teachings with me for life!

To all the **teachers and staff** who have passed through my academic life, who in one way or another have contributed to changing our university.

SUMMARY

Objective: This study aimed to assess the presence of dental caries, cariogenic diet, socioeconomic and demographic factors and oral hygiene habits in adolescents in the city of Recife - PE. **Methodology**: A cross-sectional, qualitative study was carried out, using as a research instrument a data collection form consisting of socioeconomic characterisation, oral hygiene and dietary habits and a clinical form consisting of demographic factors and the patient's dental condition. A convenience sample of 10 patients from the hebiatrics clinic of a military dental service, aged between 13 and 16 of both sexes, was used. The survey data was imported into SPSS version 23 and analysed using inferential statistical techniques (Fisher's exact test, Mann-Whitney test and Kruskal-Wallis test). **Results**: 60% of the patients analysed had dental caries. The percentage of patients without caries was 40%, of whom the percentage was higher in males. Those surveyed who had a family income of between 3 and 4 minimum wages and more than 4 to 7 minimum wages had an average dental caries rate of 0.60 and 1.20, respectively. The increase in the average number of decayed teeth was higher among those with 4 residents in the house (1.17) than among those with 5 to 6 residents in the house (0.50); among those who owned their own home rather than rented (1.14 x 0.33) and among those who brushed three times a day rather than twice a day (1.00 x 0.67). Dental caries decreased as the respondent consumed more sugar (0.33) and increased as the respondent flossed more frequently (1.67). **Conclusions**: The frequency of dental caries among the adolescents studied was high and there was no significant association between socioeconomic, demographic, oral hygiene and dietary variables and the presence of dental caries.

Keywords: Dental caries.Epidemiology.Cariogenic diet.

SUMMARY

CHAPTER 1

INTRODUCTION

Caries disease is characterised as an imbalance in the process of demineralisation and remineralisation, resulting from bacterial accumulation and metabolism on the tooth surface. With the emergence of new concepts regarding this disease, detection, especially in its early stages, has become an increasingly complex process (ALENCAR, et al. 2016).

The caries process and its implications for oral health have been of great concern to professionals in the field of dentistry. Despite being a study carried out all over the world, Gonçalves, Peres and Marcenes (2002) observed that most research focuses on school-age children, and there is not enough data in the literature on the prevalence of dental caries in adolescents.

According to Brasil (1988), the first nationwide data on the epidemiology of dental caries in adolescents in Brazil was obtained for the 15-19 age group in 1986. This survey covered the urban areas of 16 Brazilian state capitals and showed a very high DMFT index (12.69) in this age group.

Health education has to start from childhood, because the concept of health, the importance of maintaining it for general health and preventive habits tend to extend into adulthood, which means that young people without information have a high chance of becoming toothless adults with low levels of quality of life (COOLIDGE et al., 2011).

Garbin et al. (2009) reported that adolescence is considered to be a period of greater risk behaviour for dental caries, due to poor plaque control and reduced oral hygiene care, aggravated by greater independence in relation to the consumption of a more sugary diet. On the other hand, adolescence is also the phase in which young people can learn about positive attitudes and behaviours that will persist in the future, representing a fundamental moment for health promotion (RUZANY; SZWARCWALD, 2000).

The adverse effects of dental caries can influence the general development of children and adolescents, as well as the performance of their daily activities. The presence of pain, infections, early tooth loss and masticatory disorders restrict the consumption of an adequate diet and affect growth, learning, communication and recreational and leisure activities (OLIVEIRA et al., 2013). In addition to these biological effects, the literature has shown that dental caries interferes with psychological aspects associated with the self-esteem of children and adolescents. Research carried out with students aged between 11 and 14 found a significant association between dental caries and a negative impact on quality of life, especially in terms of emotional and social well-being (FERNANDES et al., 2013).

Given the disparity in access to health care, the challenge of maintaining good habits and lifestyles in order to prevent worsening oral health conditions is great, especially dietary habits. Young people in general have shown the same eating behaviour all over the world, even though they come from different cultures and countries, as they have already included soft drinks, fruit juice, coffee and milk with added sugar in their daily diet (FELDENS et al., 2013; GUIDO et al., 2011).

Educational programmes at school and with the family can achieve acceptance of the consumption of healthier and more regulated foods (FORNERIS et al., 2010; SACARDINA; MESSINA, 2012) and prevent, in parallel, obesity, another growing condition among young people, especially those living in rural areas (FRISBEE et al., 2010) and the occurrence of dental caries, since, according to Harada et al. (2005) and Freddo et al. (2008), the consumption of a cariogenic diet has been inversely proportional to the demand for dental care.

Research by Marmot (2005) has shown the relationship between socioeconomic position and health conditions. Individuals who occupy a higher position in the social hierarchy have better health conditions than those in immediately lower positions. Access to and use of dental services is also related to socioeconomic inequalities, one of the main barriers, both collectively and individually. Although there is an increase in the use of dental services in all social strata in Brazil, this use is still very unequal, as the proportion of people who have never visited dental services is eight times higher among the poorest (PERES et al., 2012).

In this context, this study aims to determine whether there is a relationship between dental caries, cariogenic diet and socioeconomic, demographic profile and oral hygiene habits in adolescents dependent on military personnel in the city of Recife - PE.

CHAPTER 2

LITERATURE REVIEW

Gonçalves, Peres and Marcenes (2002) carried out a cross-sectional study to find out the prevalence and severity of dental caries, as well as dental treatment needs, and to test their association with socioeconomic variables in 18-year-old male enlistees in the Brazilian Army. The results showed that the prevalence of caries was 81 per cent and the average DMFT index was 4.6. They observed that the higher prevalence of caries attacks was associated with the lower level of schooling of the mothers and fathers of the enlisted men, as well as the fact that the lower income and lower schooling groups concentrate most of the untreated disease and should receive priority preventive and care actions.

Baldani et al. (2002), when analysing socioeconomic factors related to dental caries, found that the etiology of social inequalities, such as poor income distribution, unemployment, technological backwardness in some sectors and high illiteracy rates, contribute to an increase in the rate of dental caries. In addition to difficulties in accessing dental services, people with different income levels are also at a disadvantage in terms of the occurrence of oral health problems.

Research by Brasil (2004) showed that caries rates among adolescents were higher than in childhood, with a significant increase in the disease during a critical period of transition to adulthood. However, the increase in the DMFT index among young people, if left unchecked, can progress into old age, with an increase in the number of lost teeth. In this sense, identifying the social and individual determinants of dental caries among adolescents can contribute to caries prevention and oral health promotion.

Mello and Antunes (2004) compared the prevalence of caries in children living in the urban and rural areas of a municipality in the state of São Paulo and found that rural schoolchildren had a higher prevalence of caries. They attributed this difference to unequal socioeconomic conditions and use of health services between urban and rural areas.

Gushi et al. (2005) carried out a cross-sectional study with data from the epidemiological survey of the State of São Paulo, Brazil, 2002, with the aim of verifying the experience of dental caries in 1,825 adolescents aged 15 to 19. The Significant Caries Index was used to define one third of the individuals with the greatest caries experience. The prevalence of caries was 90.4 per cent. There was a higher caries-free percentage in municipalities with fluoridated water. Males had the worst caries status and non-whites had the highest percentage of decayed and lost teeth. They concluded that knowledge of the distribution of caries in adolescents, identifying the risk group in this age group, as well as the need for treatment, can help prioritise the use of resources, which are always short of what is needed.

Narvai et al. (2006) carried out a study on dental caries in Brazil in relation to decline, polarisation, inequity and social exclusion, with the aim of analysing the evolution of the experience of dental caries among Brazilian schoolchildren from 1980 to 2003 and determining the distribution of caries and the access of this population to treatment for the disease. They observed a significant decline in DMFT over the study period, with the most plausible explanatory hypothesis being increased access to fluoridated water and toothpaste and changes in collective oral health programmes.

Frias et al. (2007) carried out a study with the aim of describing the prevalence of untreated dental caries in adolescents in Brazil and analysing the association of caries with individual and contextual factors in the municipalities where they live. They used a database generated by the Ministry of Health (Projeto SB - Brasil) which included information using the DMFT index for 16,833 adolescents aged between 15 and 19. The results showed that being black or brown and living in a rural area were individual determinants of a greater likelihood of having untreated caries. On the other hand, being a student was identified as a protective factor. Therefore, these results showed that there is inequality in the distribution of health services in the different Brazilian regions.

Moreira et al. (2007) carried out a study with adolescents from public and public schools, aged between 12 and 15, to check the prevalence of caries. They found that the prevalence of caries among public school students was 51.6 per cent, while among adolescents in public schools it was 9.3 per cent. A statistical test using the DMFT index showed that, with the exception of the number of decayed and missing teeth in public schools, there were significant differences between the ages studied for all the variables.

Umesi-Koleoso and Ayanbadejo (2007) administered a questionnaire to adolescents in Nigeria on oral hygiene practices, frequency and professional attitude. After collecting the data, they found that the majority of adolescents brushed their teeth once a day, and individuals belonging to the higher income social class brushed their teeth more times a day compared to individuals belonging to the lower income social class.

Kikwilu, Frencken and Mulder (2008), using a questionnaire applied to 978 patients in Tanzania, assessed the use of toothpaste and the amount of fluoride it contained. They found that urban residents were five times more likely to use toothpaste than rural residents. Proportionately, the most educated were from urban areas. These findings indicate that urban residents were better informed than rural residents about the importance of brushing with toothpaste, and imply that encouragement is needed to increase toothpaste use in rural areas. More educated respondents were more likely to brush their teeth with toothpaste compared to less educated respondents, results which indicate that education improves the oral hygiene habits of the population.

Peres et al. (2008) carried out research into the prevalence of dental caries (DMFT) and the differences in terms of gender and geographical location and found that the greater concentration of public health services in urban areas compromises and hinders the access of the population living in rural areas to dental care and it is believed that these individuals may represent an important concentration point for oral health problems. Thus, geographical location interfered with the oral health conditions of the population, and there were no differences between the genders.

Viana et al. (2009) carried out a cross-sectional prevalence study with the aim of outlining the epidemiological profile of dental caries in male enlistees aged between 17 and 19, according to an analysis of the DMFT index, its components and socioeconomic indicators. The prevalence of caries was 88.8 per cent and the average DMFT index was 5.16 ± 0.17. The results indicated statistically significant differences in the mean DMFT index, with the worst indicators being found in the groups with lower levels of schooling, lower income and from public schools, demonstrating a greater need for preventive and care measures for these groups.

According to Tseveenjav et al. (2009), education is associated with higher brushing frequency; individuals with a higher level of schooling and better socioeconomic status brush their teeth more and the highest percentage of fluoride toothpaste users belong to the highest income group.

With the aim of assessing the contribution of socioeconomic and behavioural variables in a rural population, Saliba et al. (2010) recorded a DMFT index of around three among Brazilian adolescents aged 11 to 14 and almost six among young people aged 15 to 19. They pointed out that the scarcity of epidemiological studies on the Brazilian population may compromise information on oral health, especially among rural residents. For these people, access to public services in general, schools, hospitals and health units can be difficult due to the distance from their properties and the precariousness of transport services. These and other factors, such as the lack of water treatment, sewage and rubbish collection systems, can compromise the health of this population. They concluded that unlike the municipality's urban population, which benefits from the addition of fluoride to the water supply, the rural population consumes non-fluoridated water from shallow wells dug on the properties.

Brazil (2011), comparing DMFT at the age of 12 (the index age used internationally to make comparisons), this index showed an average of 2.1, 25% lower than that found in 2003 (2.8). In the component relating to untreated (decayed) teeth, the reduction was 29 per cent (1.7 to 1.2). The percentage of "caries-free" children (DMFT = 0) went from 31% in 2003 to 44% in 2010, indicating that in 12-year-olds there has been a significant reduction in the prevalence and severity of the disease associated with greater access to restorative dental services. This significant downward trend in caries and increased access to services is also replicated in adolescents (15 to 19 years old). Although the results are encouraging in national terms, the survey also showed aspects to which the public authorities should devote greater attention, indicating the need for policies aimed at equity in care, since regional differences in the prevalence and severity of caries are still marked.

Ditmyer et *al.* (2011) analysed the prevalence and severity of dental caries in youth over a period between 2001-2009 in Nevada. The study included more than 62,000 examinations of adolescents aged 13-19, using the DMFT and *SiC*. Comparisons of student data for the DMFT confirmed that caries remains a common chronic disease among young people in Nevada, with high prevalence rates. Negative trends were found across all demographics. Over time, the youngest group exhibited an increasing proportion of caries-free individuals, while a decreasing proportion was found among the oldest. As expected, the mean *SiC* was significantly higher than the DMFT within each year of the survey in the comparison groups. Using both the caries index can help highlight oral health inequalities more accurately among different population groups within the community in order to identify the need for special preventive oral health interventions in Nevada adolescents.

With the aim of estimating a possible association between dental caries and socioeconomic conditions in adolescents aged 15 to 19 with the prevalence of toothache, a cross-sectional study of secondary data was carried out using the 2003 national survey database. Data from 15,971 people was analysed, 94.88% of all interviews. The prevalence of caries was 89.08%. After adjusting for the variables, it was found that young people with one or more decayed teeth had a 2.27 times greater risk of reporting toothache than those free of decay. The prevalence of toothache was found to be associated with socioeconomic conditions and the prevalence of caries

(OLIVEIRA; BIAZEVIC; CROSATO, 2011).

Vettore et al. (2012) investigated the association between oral and general health behaviours and socioeconomic status in a population-based cross-sectional study carried out in 2009 with students from 27 Brazilian state capitals, and the relationship between health behaviours and tooth brushing in adolescents. It was observed that the frequency of tooth brushing, as well as other health-related behaviours, was associated with socioeconomic status in a different way between the sexes. Associations were observed between health-related habits and tooth brushing frequency in both sexes, but with variations according to socioeconomic status.

Frequency of brushing is associated with parents' level of education, with statistically significant differences between the various studies analysed. Adolescents whose parents had less than four years of schooling reported less frequent brushing. Among these adolescents, 22.6% reported brushing less than once a day, 59.2% once a day and only 18.2% twice a day or more (PEREIRA et al., 2013).

Silva (2013) carried out a study to analyse the prevalence of caries (DMFT>1) and high caries burden (DMFT>4) in adolescents aged between 15 and 19 in the north-eastern region of Brazil and verified their associated factors. Among the sociodemographic variables analysed, the number of assets was found to be statistically significant in both the prevalence of caries and high levels of caries. It is important to emphasise the great influence of individuals' socio-economic conditions on their oral health, since those with lower incomes and fewer assets were the ones who were directly related to the greatest chance of having a high DMFT index. Regarding the place where the appointment was made (public, private, via health insurance and others): people who had their appointment in a private service or via health insurance had a lower chance of both caries prevalence and high caries attack than those who had their appointment in a public service.

Lopes et al. (2014) through a literature review, observed that caries is associated with different risk factors and predictors and the most consolidated are: past caries experience, enamel defects, dental biofilm, diet, mother's schooling and family income. The risk factors and predictors studied are diverse and their identification is of fundamental importance for the development of targeted strategies to reduce the incidence and prevalence of caries. Among the various socio-economic components also studied were parental schooling, family income, housing data, water supply, among others. Parental schooling is a factor that has been investigated in risk groups.

The use of fluoride is an essential and fundamental public health strategy for the prevention and control of dental caries. One of the most widely used methods for maintaining a constant level of fluoride in the oral environment is fluoride toothpaste. For many low-income countries, fluoride toothpaste is probably the only viable strategy for the population to control and prevent dental caries, while cheaper alternatives, such as water fluoridation, cannot be applied due to poor infrastructure and a lack of financial and technological resources (SCABAR et al., 2014).

Fagundes et al. (2015) found in their research that adolescents using public or philanthropic services had a higher chance of dental caries when compared to those using private services/health plans. Generally, public service users belong to a poorer economic population with less access to dental care, which would explain the association found. This suggests the need to guarantee caries prevention and control and access to restorative dental treatment in the public service.

Bonotto et al. (2015) analysed adolescents to assess the influence of gender on the prevalence of dental caries and found an association between gender and oral hygiene, with boys having a higher prevalence of dental plaque (IHOS > 1) than girls (p < 0.001). In addition, they had a higher prevalence of reporting a daily brushing frequency of less than twice a day when compared to girls (p = 0.017).

A cross-sectional study carried out by Resende et al. (2015) with adolescents from a public school in Muriaré (Minas Gerais) to analyse their eating habits found that most of the adolescents had inadequate eating habits, such as a high consumption of foods rich in fat, sweets and soft drinks, and a low daily consumption of fruit, vegetables, milk and dairy products. In addition, they observed a high rate of main meals being replaced by snacks.

Oliveira et al. (2016) studied the use of computer and television screens, consumption of meals and snacks by Brazilian adolescents and noted that this habit was higher among adolescents from public schools. This may be related to their parents' level of education and work routine, since family support is important for eating meals at the table and encouraging physical activity, as well as the awareness of the adolescents themselves. Computer and television screens have taken centre stage in the family environment, leading to profound changes in people's lifestyles. Traditional habits of family gatherings around the table have been replaced by modern habits of eating in front of screens, leading people, in general, not to pay attention to what they are eating and not to chew properly.

Adolescents from public schools and children of mothers with a higher level of education (complete high school or more) eat breakfast and have meals with their parents or guardians more often. This indicates that socioeconomic status may be related to these eating behaviours, i.e. adolescents with higher socioeconomic status have healthier behaviours than those with lower socioeconomic status (BARUFALDI et al., 2016).

Filgueira et al. (2016) conducted a cross-sectional survey of 215 adolescents (15-19 years old) to estimate their oral health status and check for any impact on quality of life. With regard to oral health status, 61 patients (28.4%) were caries-free (DMFT = 0). Untreated caries lesions were observed in 74 patients (34.4%) and 65 adolescents had filled teeth (30.2%). Only 15 adolescents (7%) had a tooth lost as a result of dental caries. Most of the adolescents surveyed live with their parents, attended primary school in a public school, have mothers who have completed secondary school and their families earn between two and three minimum wages in gross monthly income. With regard to oral health-related quality of life, just over 50% of the adolescents surveyed reported difficulty in carrying out at least one daily activity as a result of dental problems, thus showing an impact on their quality of life.

Borges et al. (2016) conducted a survey of students in southern Brazil and analysed that those living in rural areas of the municipality were 25% more likely to develop dental caries (DMFT£1) compared to those living in urban areas. Students attending municipal or state schools were five times more likely to develop dental caries compared to those in public schools. Students with mothers whose schooling was only up to 4th grade were twice as likely to develop tooth decay compared to children of mothers who had more schooling. However, students with mothers who had completed secondary school were approximately 81 per cent more likely to develop tooth decay compared to students whose mothers had completed higher education.

CHAPTER 3

OBJECTIVES

3.1 GENERAL OBJECTIVE

To assess the presence of dental caries in adolescents attending a military dental service in the city of Recife - PE.

3.2 SPECIFIC OBJECTIVES

1. To verify the cariogenic diet, socioeconomic and demographic factors and oral hygiene habits of adolescents dependent on military personnel in the city of Recife, Pernambuco.

2. To see if there is an association between socioeconomic and demographic variables and oral hygiene and eating habits with the presence of dental caries.

3.3 HYPOTHESIS

The hypothesis of this study is that dental caries will be low in the population studied.

CHAPTER 4

METHODOLOGY

4.1 Ethical considerations

In accordance with the Guidelines and Regulatory Norms for Research Involving Human Beings, through Resolution 466/12 of the National Health Council, a Free and Informed Consent Form (APPENDIX A) was drawn up containing all the information that was presented to the participants about the research and an Assent Form for minors (APPENDIX B), as well as the interviewee also receiving a Confidentiality Form (APPENDIX C), in which it is ensured that all data that identifies the research subject remains anonymous. In order to carry out this study, it was necessary to sign a Letter of Consent (APPENDIX I) from the institution involved. The project was submitted to the Research Ethics Committee of the University of Pernambuco and approved on 16/09/2016 (ANNEX II).

4.2 Study design

This was a cross-sectional, qualitative study, as it sought to gain a deeper understanding of the subjective aspects of the group studied, using a form (APPENDIX D) as a data collection tool (MOLINA, DIAS and MOLINA, 2003).

4.3 Location of the study

This study was carried out in the hebiatrics clinic of a military dental service in the city of Recife, a Brazilian municipality, capital of the state of Pernambuco, located in the north-eastern region of the country and with an area of 218 km^2 and an estimated population of 1,617,183 million inhabitants (WIKIPEDIA, 2016).

4.4 Study population

The population was made up of young adolescents dependent on military personnel of both genders, aged between 13 and 16, from the hebiatrics clinic of a military dental service in the city of Recife - PE.

4.5 Sample size and selection

A convenience sample of 10 adolescents was used to serve as a basis for future studies. Convenience sampling consists of selecting a sample from the population that is accessible, i.e. the individuals employed in this research are selected because they are readily available, not because they have been selected by means of a statistical criterion. Generally, this convenience represents greater operational ease and low sampling costs (OCHOA, 2015).

4.5.1 Inclusion criteria

- Patients within the age range;
- No braces;
- Authorisation from parents and/or guardians in the Free and Informed Consent Form;
- Consent form for minors.

4.5.2 Exclusion criteria

- Patients outside the age range;
- Patients undergoing orthodontic treatment;
- Parents and/or guardians who refuse to take part in the research or refuse to sign the Informed Consent Form;
- Adolescents who refuse to take part in the research or refuse to sign the consent form.

4.6 Calibration and diagnostic criteria

In order to obtain uniform standards for the epidemiological examination of oral health, a calibration was carried out at the FOP's Primary Care Clinic, where all the criteria adopted for the diagnosis of the "C" component of the DMFT index, according to the criteria recommended by the World Health Organisation (WHO) in its fourth version (1997), were observed with the author of the research during the month of August 2016.

4.6.1 Diagnostic criteria

The criteria used to obtain the "C" component (decayed) were those proposed by the WHO (1997). The codes for permanent dentition are shown below:

0 - <u>Healthy crown</u>:

There is no evidence of caries. Early stages of the disease are not taken into account. The following signs should be coded as healthy:

- Whitish spots;

- Discolourations or rough spots resistant to pressure from the CPI probe;

- Enamel grooves and fissures that are stained but do not show visual signs of a softened base, socketed enamel or softening of the walls, detectable with the CPI probe;

- Dark, shiny, hard and cracked areas of enamel on a tooth with moderate or severe fluorosis;

- Lesions that, based on their distribution or history, or tactile/visual examination, are the result of abrasion.

Note: All questionable lesions should be coded as a healthy tooth.

1 - Caries crown:

A groove, fissure or smooth surface has an obvious cavity, or softened tissue at the base, or enamel or wall discolouration, or there is a temporary restoration (except glass ionomer). The CPI probe should be used to confirm visual evidence of caries on the occlusal, buccal and lingual surfaces. If in doubt, the tooth should be considered healthy.

Note: In the presence of a cavity caused by caries, even if there is no disease at the time of the examination, the FSP-USP adopts the decision rule of considering the tooth to be attacked by caries and recording it as decayed.

However, this epidemiological approach does not imply that there is a need for restoration.

Note: When the crown is completely destroyed by caries, **with only the root** remaining, **the WHO recommends that code "1" be recorded only in the caseia** corresponding to the crown.

2 - Crown restored, but decayed:

There are one or more restorations and, at the same time, one or more areas are decayed. There is no distinction between primary and secondary caries, i.e. whether or not the lesions are in physical association with the restoration(s).

4.7 Research Instrument and Data Collection

At first, initial contact was made with the patient, parent and/or guardian, explaining the purpose of the research, its objective, the relevance of the study and then asking for the interviewee's participation and for the parent/guardian to sign the Free and Informed Consent Form and the Assent Form.

Secondly, an interview was carried out, in which the researcher used the cross-examination method, conducting the questions using a form. Data collection consisted of three stages. The first concerned the general identification of the patient and demographic aspects (age, gender and ethnicity) contained in the clinical file (APPENDIX E). The second stage included investigations into socio-economic aspects and oral hygiene and eating habits. The form contained 12 closed and open questions, which were applied to the study participants. Part of the questions were adapted from the socio-economic form on oral health from the SB Brasil 2000 Project (RIGO, 2010) and the rest were designed for the purposes of this study. In a third stage, data was collected from the patients through an intraoral physical examination to determine the "C" (decayed) component of the DMFT index, using sets consisting of a flat mouth mirror and a blunt-tipped exploratory probe, both sterile, and the researcher wearing the appropriate Personal Protective Equipment (PPE) for the work environment, following the Ministry of Health's biosafety standards for epidemiological surveys. For the physical examination, the patient was seated in the dental chair and the dental examination was carried out using artificial lighting (reflector) after drying the teeth with a triple syringe. The data was recorded at the time of the examination on a specific clinical form containing data relating to the patient's dental condition, in order to allow for greater reliability and veracity of the information, thus avoiding memory failure and/or distortions of the information collected.

4.8 Variables analysed

4.8.1   **Dependent variables**

> Dental caries (component "C" of the DMFT index)

4.8.2   **Independent variables**

1. DEMOGRAPHICS

> Gender

> Age

> Ethnicity

2. SOCIO-ECONOMIC

> Number of people living at home

> Housing

> Mother's occupation

> Father's occupation

> Family income

> Car ownership

3. ORAL HYGIENE AND EATING HABITS

> Frequency of tooth brushing

> Frequency of sugar consumption

> Sources of fluoride used

> Frequency of flossing

> Amount of toothpaste used as a child

> Amount of toothpaste used as a teenager

4.9 Analysing data

The data was analysed descriptively using absolute and percentage frequencies for the categorical variables and mean and standard deviation for the numerical variables, and inferentially using statistical tests. Fisher's exact test was used to assess the association between two categorical variables; the Mann-Whitney test was used to compare the number of decayed teeth between two categories and the Kruskal-Wallis test was used to compare three or more categories.

The margin of error used in deciding the statistical tests was 5.0%. The programme used to enter the data and make the statistical calculations was SPSS

version 23.

25

CHAPTER 5

RESULTS

The average family income of those surveyed was 4.14 minimum wages, with a standard deviation of 1.07 and a median of 3.75 minimum wages.

Table 1 shows the results of the socio-economic and demographic characteristics, highlighting that: the frequencies of the 4 ages (13 to 16 years) surveyed ranged from 1 to 4 adolescents; half had an income of between 3 and 4 minimum wages and the other half had an income of more than 4 to 7 minimum wages. The majority (70.0%) were white, one brown and the other two black; 60.0% of the sample had 4 residents at home, three had 5 residents at home and one had 6. The highest percentage (70.0%) lived in their own home and the other three in rented accommodation; nine mothers were housewives and one was a shop manager. All the fathers were military personnel, only one family member had no car, 60.0% had one car and three had two cars.

Table 1 - Socio-economic and demographic characteristics

Variable	n	%
TOTAL	**10**	**100,0**
Age		
13 years	4	40,0
14 years old	3	30,0
15 years	1	10,0
16 years old	2	20,0
Family income (minimum wage)		
Between 3 and 4	5	50,0
More than 4 to 7	5	50,0
Ethnicity		
White	7	70,0
Brown	1	10,0
Black	2	20,0

Variable	n	%
Number of people living at home		
4	6	60,0
5	3	30,0
6	1	10,0
Villa		
Own	7	70,0
Rented	3	30,0
Mother's occupation		
Home	9	90,0
Shop manager	1	10,0
Father's occupation		
Military	10	100,0
Car ownership		
None	1	10,0
Own a car	6	60,0
Owns two cars	3	30,0

Table 2 shows that the majority (70.0%) reported brushing three times a day and the other three brushed twice a day. The frequencies of those who consumed sugar once a day, twice a day and three times a day were 3, 4 and 3 respectively. All used fluoride professionally, 70.0% as a gel, 10.0% as a mouthwash and 20.0% in both forms. The frequencies of those who didn't floss, flossed once or twice were 4, 3 and 3 respectively.

Table 2 - Evaluation of oral hygiene habits and diet variables

Variable	n	%
TOTAL	**10**	**100,0**
Frequency of tooth brushing		
Twice a day	3	30,0
Three times a day	7	70,0
Frequency of sugar consumption in the diet		
Once a day	3	30,0
Twice a day	4	40,0
Three times a day	3	30,0
Use of professional fluoride		
In gel form	7	70,0
Mouthwash	1	10,0
Both forms	2	20,0
Frequency of flossing		
Not once	4	40,0
Once a day	3	30,0
Twice a day	3	30,0
Amount of toothpaste used as a child		
Photo 1	1	10,0
Photo 2	1	10,0
Photo 3	4	40,0
Photo 4	4	40,0
Amount of toothpaste used as a teenager		

Photo 1   -   -
Photo 2   1   10,0
Photo 3   2   20,0
Photo 4   7   70,0

The number of decayed teeth ranged from 0 to 3, with a mean of 0.90, a standard deviation of 0.99 and a median of 1.00 tooth.

Table 3 shows that 4 adolescents had no tooth decay; 4 had one cavity. The frequencies of those with two and three cavities were one each. It can be seen that 60.0% had dental caries and 40.0% did not.

Table 3 - Assessment of dental caries

riablen	Va	%
TAL10	**TO**	**100,0**
Number of teeth with caries		
e4	Non	40,0
4	One	40,0
o1	Tw	10,0
ee1	Thr	10,0
Dental caries		
m6	Co	60,0
4	Sem	40,0

Table 4 shows the results of the study of the association between dental caries and each of the socioeconomic, demographic, oral hygiene habits and diet variables. Although some percentage frequencies with caries showed high differences for the margin of error set (5%), there was no significant difference (p > 0.05) between the presence or absence of caries and the socioeconomic, demographic, oral hygiene habits and diet variables.

Table 4 - Presence or absence of caries according to socioeconomic and demographic variables, oral hygiene habits and diet

Variable	Dental caries		TOTAL	p-value
	Yes	No		

	n	%	n	%	n	%
TOTAL	6	60,0	4	40,0	10	100,0
Gender						$p^{(1)} = 0.190$
Male	1	25,0	3	75,0	4	100,0
Female	5	83,3	1	16,7	6	100,0
Number of residents at home -						$p^{(1)} = 1,000$
4 people	4	66,7	2	33,3	6	100,0
5 or 6 people	2	50,0	2	50,0	4	100,0
Villa						$p^{(1)} = 0.500$
Own	5	71,4	2	28,6	7	100,0
Rented	1	33,3	2	66,7	3	100,0
Family income (minimum wage)						$p^{(1)} = 1,000$
Between 3 and 4	3	60,0	2	40,0	5	100,0
More than 4 to 7	3	60,0	2	40,0	5	100,0
Frequency of tooth brushing						$p^{(1)} = 1,000$
Twice a day	2	66,7	1	33,3	3	100,0
Three times a day	4	57,1	3	42,9	7	100,0
Frequency of sugar consumption in the diet						$p^{(1)} = 0.743$
Once a day	2	66,7	1	33,3	3	100,0
Twice a day	3	75,0	1	25,0	4	100,0
Three times a day	1	33,3	2	66,7	3	100,0
Frequency of flossing						$p^{(1)} = 0.400$
Not once	2	50,0	2	50,0	4	100,0
Twice a day	1	33,3	2	66,7	3	100,0
Three times a day	3	100,0	-	-	3	100,0

(1) Using Fisher's exact test.

There were no significant differences ($p > 0.05$) between the categories in terms of the number of cavities; however, it is worth noting that the average number of cavities was correspondingly higher among the female respondents than the male respondents (1.17 x 0.50); among those who had 4 residents at home than among those who had 5 to 6 residents at home (1.17 x 0.50); among those who owned their own home rather than rented (1.14 x 0.33); among those with a family income of more than 4 to 7 minimum wages rather than those with a family income of between 3 and 4 minimum wages (1.20 x 0.60); among those who brushed three times rather than twice a day (1.00 x 0.67). Dental caries decreased as the respondent consumed more sugar; it increased as the respondent flossed more frequently, according to the results shown in Table 5.

Table 5 - Statistics on the number of decayed teeth according to socioeconomic and demographic variables and oral hygiene and dietary habits

Variable	Average	Standard deviation	p-value
Sex			
Male (n = 4)	0,50	1,00	$p^{(1)} = 0.243$
Female (n = 6)	1,17	0,98	
No. of residents at home			
4 (n = 6)	1,17	1,17	$p^{(1)} = 0.438$
5 to 6 (n = 4)	0,50	0,58	
Villa			
Own (n = 7)	1.14	1,07	$p^{(1)} = 0.400$
Rented (n = 3)	0,33	0,58	
Family income (minimum wage)			
Between 3 and 4 (n = 5)	0,60	0,55	$p^{(1)} = 0.683$
More than 4 to 7 (n = 5)	1,20	1,30	
Frequency of tooth brushing			
Twice a day (n = 3)	0,67	0,58	$p^{(1)} = 1.00$
Three times a day (n = 7)	1,00	1,16	
Frequency of sugar consumption in the diet			
Once a day (n = 3)	1,33	1,53	$p^{(2)} = 0.475$
Twice a day (n = 4)	1,00	0,82	
Three times a day (n = 3)	0,33	0,58	
Frequency of flossing			
Not once (n = 4)	0,50	0,58	$p^{(2)} = 0.286$
Once a day (n = 3)	0,67	1,16	
Twice a day (n = 3)	1,67	1,15	

(1) Using the Mann-Whitney test
(2) Using the Kruskal-Wallis test.

CHAPTER 6

DISCUSSION

This study involved 10 adolescents who were accompanied by their parents during the clinical examination. As this was a convenience sample, no probabilistic population inference conclusions will be presented for the municipality, but the results presented should serve as a basis for future more comprehensive and conclusive studies. During data collection, everyone who was asked to take part cooperated, and there was no opposition to it. However, many difficulties were encountered in relation to the working hours of the professional who attended the adolescent at the clinic, as well as a high number of patient absences, which hampered the size of the sample studied.

The caries process and its implications for oral health have been a major concern for dental professionals. In the results found in this study, there was a small age range from 13 to 16 years old, and due to the number of absentees, it was not possible to obtain more data to enrich the study. Although this is a worldwide study, this lack of data is also confirmed by Gonçalves, Peres and Marcenes (2002), who noted that the majority of research focuses on school-age children and that there is not enough data in the literature on the prevalence of dental caries in adolescents. In addition, the epidemiological studies carried out on adolescents, both in Brazil and in developed countries, lack uniformity in terms of diagnostic criteria and sampling procedures, which makes it difficult to establish comparisons of research at this age (GUSHI, et al., 2005).

Of the total number of people surveyed with dental caries, more than half had decayed teeth. Fagundes et al. (2015) explained this association, revealing that public service users belong to an economically poorer population with less access to dental care, suggesting the need to guarantee caries prevention and control and access to restorative dental treatments in the public service. Despite the recognised importance of oral health, a significant portion of the Brazilian population does not use dental services frequently (GIBILINI et al., 2016).

According to the results obtained, the number of cavities was higher in families with higher incomes (more than 4 to 7 minimum wages), diverging from the results found by Silva (2013), who reported that those with lower incomes and fewer assets were more likely to have a high rate of cavities. One possible reason for this difference could be that parents don't inspect their children's oral hygiene, believing that they do it correctly and every day, without needing to be reprimanded or taught.

In this study, skin colour had no impact on quality of life. Contradicting this, Gushi et al. (2005) reported that non-whites had a higher percentage of decayed and missing teeth. Similarly, being black or brown and living in a rural area were individual determinants of a greater likelihood of having untreated caries (FRIAS et al., 2007). Further research is needed with more adolescents dependent on the military in order to add results to the data collected, with the aim of justifying the studies by the aforementioned authors.

In relation to the results found, it was observed that dental caries was higher in the presence of fewer residents living at home, diverging from the studies carried out by Melo et al. (2011), in which they found that living in households with six or more residents, more than three people per room and living in the area for three or more years were statistically associated with the experience of dental caries. One of the most likely justifications found for this result is that nowadays the number of children, however small, has no effect on reducing the presence of caries.

With regard to the occupation of the parents observed in this study, the majority of the mothers were housewives (90%) and the fathers were military personnel, so we could assume that the mothers spent more time with their children at home and could supervise and teach them better mouth brushing and cariogenic diet control. Daily brushing practices and diet control are important oral health precautions. In the vast majority of families, the process of acquiring oral hygiene habits begins early in childhood, but with the social problems encountered by some families, this attitude sometimes goes unnoticed by those responsible, who should at least carry out the first brushing sessions for their children, and in many cases, children imitate the actions carried out by their elders (MODENA, 2005).

Analysing the results of the survey, it was noted that tooth decay increased among those who brushed their teeth more often a day and decreased as sugar consumption increased. We can justify this behavioural analysis by the high exposure to screens among students from public schools. This may be due to the fact that public school students have more access to technological advances, such as electrical and electronic equipment, and therefore spend more time using this equipment (Oliveira et al., 2010). Another contributing factor is the strong influence of the media on eating behaviour. Industries invest heavily in fast-food adverts, high-calorie foods, carbonated drinks, sugary breakfast cereals and other ultra-processed products, which can have an impact on the formation of eating habits that risk the development of chronic diseases in children and adolescents (MOURA, 2010).

The use of fluoride is fundamental in the prevention and control of dental caries. One of the most widely used methods for maintaining a constant level of fluoride in the oral environment is fluoride toothpaste (SCABAR et al., 2014). With regard to its use, the highest percentage (70%) found in the survey was professional fluoride in gel form, and there were no respondents who did not use fluoride sources.

In many low-income countries, fluoride toothpaste is probably the best way for the population to control and prevent dental caries (SCABAR et al., 2014). From the data researched regarding the amount of toothpaste used as a child and adolescent, it was found that when it came to the amount, there was a prevalence for completely filling the bristles of the brushes, which cannot be reiterated in the research carried out by Evans (1991). It is assumed that the parents of the children seen at the clinic did not supervise or participate in brushing their children's teeth, believing that they brushed their teeth correctly, or that the parents did not understand how much toothpaste was needed, with some parents explaining that the reason for their lack of participation at home was due to work or even not knowing the correct brushing techniques. It is important to emphasise that many of them have not received this information, so it is wrong to demand habits that have not been passed down from past generations. The reality of this population's life is of great importance in determining their health habits (BRASIL, 2006).

Resistance to flossing is observed among young people. They find it difficult to use because of the skill required, as it requires training, and they are lazy to adopt it as a routine resource (FLORES; DREHMER, 2003). The data obtained in the survey emphasises that 40% of respondents do not use dental floss and 30% use it at least twice a day. These findings were also similar in another study in which only 20% used dental floss regularly (DARBY et al., 2012).

Analyses carried out with adolescents to assess the influence of gender on the prevalence of dental caries found an association between gender and oral hygiene, with boys having a higher prevalence of dental plaque than girls (p< 0.001). In addition, they had a higher prevalence of reporting a daily brushing frequency of less than twice a day when compared to girls (BONOTTO et al.,2015). In contrast to these analyses, the highest number of caries in this study is represented by females. Adolescence is a stage of great risk for oral health problems such as caries, gingivitis, recession and gingival bleeding. Sociodemographic and psychosocial factors and the lifestyle adopted by the individual determine hygiene habits and their own health (JÚNIOR et al., 2016).

Adolescence is a phase of life marked by processes of vulnerability and definition, as well as social insertion in search of autonomy (ASSIS; AVANCI 2015). It is important to emphasise to adolescents the importance of oral hygiene care: correct brushing, flossing, the precise amount of toothpaste and the presence of parents to understand the importance of good oral education. The dental surgeon plays a significant role in motivating self-care at this stage, as it is common for adolescents to neglect oral hygiene care, adopt a more cariogenic diet and omit dental appointments.

Over the last three decades, globalisation has established new paradigms and profound changes in food choices. This scenario, combined with the increased use of television and other screens such as video games and computers by children and adolescents, jeopardises the adoption of a healthy lifestyle. The distraction caused by televisions interferes with the physiological signals of hunger and satiety, leading to inadequate food choices with excessive consumption of high-calorie, low-nutrient products (BICKHAM et al., 2013).

In this context, further research is needed to confirm the frequency and factors related to dental caries in the population studied.

CHAPTER 7

CONCLUSIONS

According to the results found, it can be concluded that:

- The frequency of dental caries among adolescents was high;

- Sugar consumption and socioeconomic factors were high, as were oral hygiene habits;

- Dental caries was higher among females;

- There was no significant association between socioeconomic and demographic variables, oral hygiene habits and diet and the presence of dental caries;

- The hypothesis of this study was not accepted.

CHAPTER 8

BIBLIOGRAPHICAL REFERENCES

ALENCAR, A.A. et al. Alternative caries detection methods: a literature review.**Jornada Odontológica dos Acadêmicos da Católica**, v. 1, 2016.

ASSIS, S.G ; AVANCI, J.Q.Adolescence and collective health: between risk and youth protagonism. **Ciênc. Saúde Colet**, v. 20, n.11, p. 231-238, 2015.

BALDANI, M.H. et al. Dental caries and socioeconomic conditions in the State of Paraná, Brazil, 1996. **Cad. Saúde Pública**, v. 18, n. 3, p. 755-763, 2002.

BARUFALDI, L. A. et al. ERICA: prevalence of healthy eating behaviours in Brazilian adolescents. **Revista de SaúdePública**, v.50, n.1, p. 6, 2016.

BICKHAM, D.S. et al. Characteristics of screen media use associated with higher BMI in young adolescents. **Pediatrics**, v. 131, n. 5, p. 935-941, 2013.

BONOTTO, D.M.V. et al. Dental caries and gender in adolescents. **Revista da Faculdade de Odontologia-UPF**, v. 20, n. 2, 2015.

BORGES, T.S. et al. Factors associated with caries: a survey of students in southern Brazil. **Revista Paulista de Pediatria**, v. 34, n. 4, p. 489-494, 2016.

BRAZIL. Ministry of Health - Oral Health Division. **Epidemiological Survey of Oral Health: Brazil - urban area**. 1986. Series C: studies and projects, 1988.

BRAZIL. Ministry of Health. Health Care Secretariat. Primary Care Department. **SB Brasil 2003 Project: oral health conditions of the Brazilian population 2002-2003**. Main Results. Brasilia, 2004.

BRAZIL - Ministry of Health. Health Care Secretariat. **Department of Primary Care.** Saúde Bucal/Ministério da Saúde, Secretaria de Atenção à Saúde- Brasília: MS,2006.

BRAZIL. Ministry of Health. **SB Brasil Project 2010 - National Oral Health Survey.** Main results 2010. Brasília; 2011.

COOLIDGE, T. et al. Thinking about going to the dentist: a Contemplation Ladder to assess dentally-avoidant individuals' readiness to go to a dentist. **BMC oral health**, v. 11, n. 1, p. 1, 2011.

DARBY, l. et al. Periodontal health of dental clients in a community health setting. **Australian dental journal**, v. 57, n. 4, p. 486-492, 2012.

DITMYER, M. et al. Inequalities of caries experience in Nevada youth expressed by DMFT index vs. Significant Caries Index (SiC) over time. **BMC Oral Health**, v.11, n.12, p. 01-10, 2011.

EVANS, D. J. A study of developmental defects in enamel in 10-year-old high social class children residing in a non-fluoridated area. **Community dental health**, v. 8, n.1, p. 31-38, 1991.

FAGUNDES, S. M. et al. Dental caries and associated factors among adolescents in the north of the state of Minas Gerais, Brazil: a hierarchical analysis. **Journal Ciência & Saúde Coletiva**, v. 20, n. 11, 2015.

FELDENS, C. A. et al. Food expenditures, cariogenic dietary practices and childhood dental caries in southern Brazil. **Caries research**, v. 47, n. 5, p. 373-381, 2013.

FERNANDES, M.L.M.F. et al. Dental caries and the need for orthodontic treatment: impact on the quality of life of schoolchildren. **Pesquisa Brasileira em Odontopediatria e Clínica Integrada**, v. 13, n. 1, 2013.

FILGUEIRA, A.C.G. et al. Oral health of school adolescents. **HOLOS**, v. 1, p.161-172, 2016.

FLORES, E. M.T.L.; DREHMER, T.M. Conhecimento, percepções, comportamentos e representações de saúde e doença bucal dos adolescentes de escolas públicas de dois bairros de Porto Alegre. **Ciência & Saúde Coletiva**, v. 8, n. 3, p. 743-752, 2003.

FORNERIS, T. et al. Results of a Rural School-Based Peer-Led Intervention for Youth: Goals for Health. **Journal of School Health**, v. 80, n. 2, p. 57-65, 2010.

FREDDO, S.L. et al. Oral hygiene habits and use of dental services among teenage students in a city in southern Brazil. **Cadernos de saude publica**, v. 24, n. 9, p. 1991-2000, 2008.

FRIAS, A. C. et al. Individual and contextual determinants of the prevalence of untreated dental caries in Brazil. **Revista Panamericana de Salud Publica**, v. 22, n. 4, p. 279-285, 2007.

FRISBEE, S.J. et al. Self-reported dental hygiene, obesity, and systemic inflammation in a paediatric rural community cohort. **BMC oral health**, v. 10, n. 1, p. 21, 2010.

GARBIN, C.A.S. et al. Oral health in the perception of adolescents. **Rev Salud Publica**, v. 11, n. 2, p. 268-277, 2009.

GIBILINI, C. et al. Access to dental services and self-perception of oral health in adolescents, adults and the elderly. **Archives of Dentistry**, v. 46, n. 4, 2016.

GONÇALVES, E. R.; PERES, M. A.; MARCENES, W. Dental caries and socio-economic conditions: a cross-sectional study of 18-year-olds in Florianópolis, Santa CATARINA, Brazil. **Cad. Saúde Pública**, Rio de Janeiro, v. 18, n.3, p. 699706, May/June, 2002.

GUIDO, J. A. et al. Caries prevalence and its association with brushing habits, water availability, and the intake of sugared beverages. **International Journal of Paediatric Dentistry**, v. 21, n. 6, p. 432-440, 2011.

GUSHI, L. L. et al. Dental caries in adolescents aged 15 to 19 in the State of São Paulo, Brazil, 2002. **Cad. Saúde Pública**, Rio de Janeiro, v. 21, n.5, p. 1383-1391, Sept./Oct., 2005.

HARADA,S. et al. Relationships between lifestyle and dental health behaviours in a rural population in Japan. **Community Dent Oral Epidemiology**, v. 33, n. 1, p. 1724, 2005.

JÚNIOR, S. et al. Adolescent Oral Health: Literature Review. **Adolesc. Saúde (Online)**, p. 95-103, 2016.

KIKWILU, E.N; FRENCKEN, J.E; MULDER, J. Utilisation of toothpaste and fluoride content in toothpaste manufactured in Tanzania. **Acta Odontologica Scandinavica**, v. 66, n. 5, p. 293-299, 2008.

LOPES, L.M. et al. Indicators and risk factors of dental caries in children in Brazil-A literature review. **Revista da Faculdade de Odontologia-UPF**, v.19, n. 2, 2014.

MARMOT, M. Historical perspective: the social determinants of disease-some blossoms. **Epidemiologic perspectives & innovations: EP+ I**, v. 2, p. 4, 2005.

MELLO, T.R.C.; ANTUNES, J.L.F. Prevalence of dental caries in schoolchildren in the rural region of Itapetininga, São Paulo, Brazil.**Cad. Saúde Pública**, v. 20, n. 3, p. 829-835, 2004.

MELO, M.M.D.C. et al. Factors associated with dental caries in preschool children in Recife, Pernambuco, Brazil. **Cad Saúde Pública**, p. 471-485, 2011.

MODENA, C.M. **Ciência e Saúde coletiva**, v.10, n.1, jan/mar., 2005.

MOLINA, A; DIAS, E.; MOLINA, A. E. **Initiation into scientific research: manual for professionals and students in the areas of health, biological sciences and humanities.** Recife: EDUPE, 2003.

MOREIRA, P.V.L. et al. Caries prevalence in adolescents from public and public schools in the city of João Pessoa, Paraíba, Brazil. **Ciência & Saúde Coletiva**, v. 12, n. 5, p. 1229-1236, 2007.

MOURA, N.C. Influence of the media on the eating behaviour of children and adolescents. **Segurança Alimentar e Nutricional**, v. 17, n. 1, p. 113-122, 2010.

NARVAI, P. C. et al. Dental caries in Brazil: decline, polarisation, inequity and social exclusion. **Rev Panam Salud Publica**, v.19, n.6, p. 385-393, 2006.

OCHOA, Carlos. **Non-probability sampling: Convenience sampling, 2015.** Available at: <https://www.netquest.com/blog/br/blog/br/amostra- conveniencia>. Accessed on: 07

Apr. 2017.

OLIVEIRA, B. A.; BIAZEVIC, M. G. H.; CROSATO, E. M. Prevalence of toothache, dental caries and socioeconomic conditions: a study in young Brazilian adults. **Odonto**, v.19, n.38, p. 07-14, 2011.

OLIVEIRA, T.C. et al. Physical activity and sedentary lifestyle in public and private schoolchildren in São Luís. **Revista de saude publica**, v. 44, n. 6, p.996- 1004, 2010.

OLIVEIRA, D.C. et al. Reported impact of oral alterations on the quality of life of adolescents: a systematic review. **Pesqui. bras. odontopediatria clín. integr**, v. 13, n. 1, 2013.

OLIVEIRA, J.S. et al. ERICA: use of screens and consumption of meals and snacks by Brazilian adolescents. **Revista de Saúde Pública**, v. 50, n. 1, p. 7, 2016.

WORLD HEALTH ORGANISATION (OMS). **Basic oral health surveys**. 4 ed, 1997.

PEREIRA, C. et al. Oral health behaviours in Portuguese adolescents. **Portuguese Journal of Public Health**, v. 31, n. 2, p. 145-152, 2013.

PERES, K.G. et al. Reduction of social inequalities in utilisation of dental care in Brazil from 1998 to 2008. **Revista de saude publica**, v. 46, n. 2, p. 250-258, 2012.

PERES, S. H. C. S. et al. Polarisation of dental caries in adolescents in the southwestern region of the State of São Paulo, Brazil. **Ciência & Saúde Coletiva**, v. 13, p. 21552162, 2008.

RESENDE, F. R. et al. Analysis of the eating habits and hygiene practices of adolescents at a public school in Muriaé (MG). **Revista científica da faminas**, v. 11, n. 1, 2015.

RIGO, L. **Dental Caries and Fluorosis in Adolescence: Prevalence and Associated Factors**. 2010. 174 f. Thesis (Doctorate in Dentistry) - Faculty of Dentistry, University of Pernambuco, Camaragibe, 2010.

RUZANY, M.H; SZWARCWALD C.L. Missed opportunities for comprehensive adolescent care: results of a pilot study. **Rev Adolescencia Latino Americana**, Porto Alegre, v.2, n 1, p.26-35, jun 2000.

SACARDINA, G.A.; MESSINA, P. Good oral health and diet. **BioMed Research International**, v. 2012, 2012.

SALIBA, N.A. et al. Dental loss in a rural population and the goals established for the World Health Organisation. **Ciencia & saude coletiva**, v. 15, p. 1857-1864, 2010.

SCABAR, L.F. et al.**Frequency of Toothpaste Use According to Income and Schooling: A Systematic Review**, São Paulo, p.318-325, 30 Jul. 2014. Available at   :
<https://www.unip.br/comunicacao/publicacoes/ics/edicoes/2014/03_jul- sep/V32_n3_2014_p318a325.pdf>. Accessed on: 15 March 2017.

SILVA, M.F.C.D.A. **Prevalence and factors associated with dental caries and high caries attack in adolescents in the northeast region of Brazil.** 2013. 23 f. TCC (Collective Health) - Aggeu Magalhães Research Centre, Recife, 2013.

TSEVEENJAV, B. et al. Patterns of oral cleaning habits and use of fluoride among dentate adults in Finland. **Oral health & preventive dentistry**, v. 8, n. 3, p. 287-294, 2009.

UMESI-KOLEOSO, D. C.; AYANBADEJO, P. O. Oral Hygiene Practices Among Adolescents In Surulere, Lagos Sate, Nigeria. **Nigerian quarterly journal of hospital medicine**, v. 17, n. 3, p. 112-115, 2007.

VETTORE, M. V. et al. Socioeconomic status, tooth brushing frequency and health behaviours in Brazilian adolescents: an analysis based on the National School Health Survey (PeNSE). **Cad. Saúde Pública**, Rio de Janeiro, v.28, p. 101-113, 2012.

VIANA, A. R. P. et al.Prevalence of dental caries and socioeconomic conditions in young enlistees from Manaus, Amazonas, Brazil. **Rev Bras Epidemiol**, p. 680-687, 2009.

WIKIPEDIA. Available at: <https://pt.wikipedia.org/wiki/Recife> Accessed on: 27 April 2016.

APPENDIX A - Informed Consent Form

We invite you to take part in the research entitled: "DENTAL CARIES, CARIOGENIC DIET, SOCIOECONOMIC AND DEMOGRAPHIC FACTORS AND ORAL HYGIENE HABITS IN ADOLESCENTS IN THE CITY OF RECIFE- PE", under the responsibility of the supervisor Prof[s] Dr[a] Silvia Regina Sampaio Bezerra de Moraes and researcher Samara Sandrelly de Moura Gomes, with the aim of finding out about the prevalence of dental caries, cariogenic diet, socioeconomic, demographic and behavioural factors in adolescents in the city of Recife, Pernambuco.

To carry out this work, we will use the following methods: your participation in this research will consist of two phases. The first will be a clinical examination to check for dental caries and the second will be the application of a form containing questions about eating habits, oral hygiene and socio-economic factors. The results of the study will be kept for two years and incinerated after this period. We would like to make it clear that, during and after the end of the study, we will keep all the data that identifies the research subject anonymous and will only use the data inherent in the development of the study to publicise it. We would also like to inform you that after the end of the study, any and all media that could identify you, such as film footage, photos, recordings, etc., will be destroyed, leaving nothing to compromise the anonymity of your participation now or in the future. The methodology used in the research may result in a small risk or minimal physical discomfort for the participant as a result of the clinical examination. If this occurs, the examination will be suspended immediately, if you so wish. Sterile material and PPE will be used for the examination in order to avoid the possibility of contamination for the participant and the researcher. The benefits expected from the results of this research are related to your participation, and will be to contribute to the development of epidemiological research into dental caries in relation to the socioeconomic and demographic reality of the

Brazilian population.

You will have the following rights: the guarantee of receiving an answer to any question or clarification to any doubt about the procedures, risks, benefits and others related to the research; the freedom to withdraw my consent at any time and stop participating in the study without this causing damage to your relationship with the researcher or the institution; the security that I will not be identified and that confidentiality of information related to my privacy will be maintained; the commitment to provide me with updated information during the study, even if this may affect my willingness to continue participating; if there are additional expenses these will be absorbed by the research budget.

If you have any questions or queries, please contact the researchers:

1) Prof³ Drª Silvia Regina Sampaio Bezerra de Moraes (**Supervisor**)

Address: Rua Serra Dourada, 51 Aldeia, Camaragibe-PE. CEP: 54789-500. Telephone: 31029143

2) Academic: Samara Sandrelly de Moura Gomes (**Researcher**)

Address: Rua Rodrigues Ferreira, 45, Várzea - PE. CEP: 50810-020. Telephone: 30348115

If your questions are not resolved by the researchers or your rights are denied, please contact the Research Ethics Committee of the University of Pernambuco, located at Av. Agamenon Magalhães, S/N, Santo Amaro, Recife-PE, telephone 81-3183-3775 or via e-mail at comite.etica@upe.br.

I ___________________________________ ,_____________________________________ the   person

responsible for

Having received all the clarifications and being aware of my rights, I agree to allow my dependent to take part in this research, as well as authorising the disclosure and publication of all information transmitted by him/her, except personal data, in publications and events of a scientific nature.

Local: C-ODONTO/PM-

PEData:___ / ___ / ___

Signature of the person
responsible   Researcher's signature

* Prepared on the basis of Resolution 466/12 of the National Health Council of the Ministry of

Health/CONEP.

APPENDIX B - Consent Form

You are invited to participate in the research entitled: "TOOTH CARIES, CARIOGENIC DIET, SOCIOECONOMIC, DEMOGRAPHIC FACTORS AND MORAL HYGIENE HABITS IN ADOLESCENTS IN THE CITY OF RECIFE- PE", under the responsibility of the supervisor Prof[s] . Dr[a] Silvia Regina Sampaio Bezerra de Moraes and researcher Samara Sandrelly de Moura Gomes with the aim of finding out about the prevalence of dental caries, cariogenic diet, socioeconomic, demographic and behavioural factors in adolescents in the city of Recife, Pernambuco.

To carry out this work, we will use the following methods: your participation in this research will consist of two phases. The first will be a clinical examination to check for dental caries and the second will be the application of a form containing questions about eating habits, oral hygiene and socio-economic factors. The results of the study will be kept for two years and incinerated afterwards. Your name and all data identifying you will be kept strictly confidential before, during and after the end of the study. The methodology used in the research may result in a small risk or minimal physical discomfort for the participant as a result of the clinical examination. If this occurs, the examination will be suspended immediately, if you so wish. Sterile material and PPE will be used for the examination in order to avoid the possibility of contamination for the participant and the researcher. The expected benefits of participating in this research will be to contribute to the development of epidemiological research into dental caries in relation to the socioeconomic and demographic reality of the Brazilian population. During the course of the research you have the following rights: the guarantee of receiving an answer to any question or clarification to any doubt about the procedures, risks, benefits and others related to the research; the freedom to withdraw my consent at any time and stop participating in the study without this causing harm to your relationship with the researcher or the institution; the security that I will not be identified and that confidentiality of information related to my privacy will be maintained; the commitment to provide me with updated information during the study, even if this may affect my willingness to continue participating; if there are additional expenses these will be absorbed by the research budget.

If you have any doubts, you should speak to your guardian so that they can contact the researchers to resolve your problem.

1)Prof[a] Dr[a] Silvia Regina Sampaio Bezerra de Moraes (**Supervisor**)

Address: Rua Serra Dourada, 51 Aldeia, Camaragibe-PE. CEP: 54789-500. Telephone: 31029143

2)Academic: Samara Sandrelly de Moura Gomes (**Researcher**)

Address:Rua Rodrigues Ferreira, 45, Várzea - PE. CEP: 50810-020. Telephone: 30348115

If your questions are not resolved by the researchers or your rights are denied, please contact the Research Ethics Committee of the University of Pernambuco, located at Av. Agamenon Magalhães, S/N, Santo Amaro, Recife-PE, telephone 81-3183-3775 or via e-mail at comite.etica@upe.br.

I_______________________________________ , having received all the clarifications and my
I have signed the ICF and agree to take part in this research.

Place: C-ODONTO/PM-PEData   : __/__/__

   Signature of the minor   Researcher's signature

* Prepared on the basis of Resolution 466/12 of the National Health Council of the Ministry of Health/CONEP.

APPENDIX C - Confidentiality Agreement

I, Prof[a] Dir* Silvia Regina Sampaio Bezerra de Moraes and undergraduate student Samara Sandrelly de Moura Gomes, hereby undertake to keep all data used for the research entitled: "TOOTH CARIES, CARIOGENIC DIET, SOCIOECONOMIC, DEMOGRAPHIC FACTORS AND MORAL HYGIENE HABITS IN ADOLESCENTS FROM THE CITY OF RECIFE- PE", during and after its conclusion.

Recife, _______//

____

Signature and stamp of the Researcher in Charge

Researcher's signature

45

APPENDIX D - Data Collection Form

1. Numero de pessoas morando em casa

2. Moradia

1. Própria
2. Própria em aquisição
3. Alugada
4. Cedida
5. Outros

3. Ocupação da mãe

____

4. Ocupação do pai

____

5. Renda familiar (em reais)

____

6. Posse de automóvel

0. Não possui
1. Possui 1 automóvel
2. Possui 2 ou mais automóveis

7. Frequência da escovação dentária:

0 - Nenhuma vez
1 - 1x ao dia
2 - 2x ao dia
3 - 3x ao dia
4 - 4x ou mais ao dia

8. Frequência do consumo de açúcar na dieta alimentar. (doces, biscoitos, bala, sobremesa...)?

0 - Nenhuma vez
1 - 1x ao dia
2 - 2x ao dia
3 - 3x ao dia ou mais
4 - 1x ou mais na semana

9. Uitiliza ou utilizou fontes de flúor (profissional) ?

0 - Nunca utilizou
1 - Aplicação de flúor em forma de gel
2 - Bochechos com flúor
3 - Ambas as fontes de flúor

10. Frequêcia do uso do fio dental:

0 - Nenhuma vez
1 - 1x ao dia
2 - 2x ao dia
3 - 3x ao dia
4 - 4x ou mais vezes por semana

11. Quantidade de creme dental usado quando criança (observe a figura a baixo):

1 2 3 4

12. Quantidade de creme dental usado quando adolescente (observe a figura a baixo):

1 2 3 4

APPENDIX E - Clinical Data Collection Form

Data:...

Nome:..

Prontuário:

Gênero   **Idade**   **Etnia** ______________________

M – Masculino

F – Feminino

Nascimento:

Dia   Mês   Ano

	18	17	16	15	14	13	12	11	21	22	23	24	25	26	27	28
Coroa																

	48	47	46	45	44	43	42	41	31	32	33	34	35	36	37	38
Coroa																

ANNEXES

ANNEX I - Letter of Consent

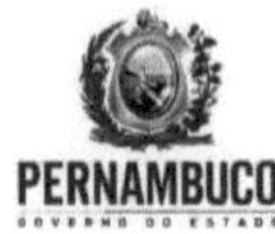

SECRETARIAT OF SOCIAL DEFENCE
MILITARY POLICE OF PERNAMBUCO
HEALTH DIRECTORATE
DENTAL CENTRE
R.Betânia, s/n° (Pça do Derby),Recife-PE CEP 52010-140
Phone: (81) 3181-1441, E-mail: codontopmpe@gmail.com

We hereby declare for all due purposes that we have agreed to receive SAMARA SANDRELLY DE MOURA GOMES, student of the 8th period of the Undergraduate Dentistry Course of the Faculty of Dentistry of the University of Pernambuco (FOP/UPE), enrolment n° 05023689425 to carry out the research of the Course Conclusion Work entitled: "TOOTH CARIES, CARIOGENIC DIET, SOCIOECONOMIC, DEMOGRAPHIC FACTORS AND MORAL HYGIENE HABITS IN ADOLESCENTS FROM THE CITY OF RECIFE- PE" at the Dental Centre of the Military Police of Pernambuco, under the guidance of Profa. Dr. Silvia Regina Sampa. Dr Silvia Regina Sampaio Bezerra de Moraes, and we undertake to keep all the data used to carry out this research strictly confidential. This project may result in a small risk or minimal physical discomfort for the participant as a result of the clinical examination. If this occurs, the examination will be suspended immediately, if you wish. Sterile material and PPE will be used for the examination to avoid the possibility of contamination for the participant and the researcher. We would like to point out that this authorisation is an ethical precondition for carrying out any study involving human beings (in any form and dimension), in line with Resolution 466/12 of the National Health Council, and without which the analysis process carried out by the Research Ethics Committee cannot be completed.

Recife, 09 June 2016.

____

Lt Col PM/QOD Ronaldo de Carvalho Raimundo

ANNEX II - Proof of Approval by the Research Ethics Committee

DETALHAR PROJETO DE PESQUISA

— DADOS DA VERSÃO DO PROJETO DE PESQUISA

Título da Pesquisa: Avaliação de cárie dentária, dieta cariogênica e fatores socioeconômicos em adolescentes dependentes de militares da cidade de Recife-PE
Pesquisador Responsável: SILVIA REGINA SAMPAIO BEZERRA
Área Temática:
Versão: 3
CAAE: 56806916.3.0000.5207
Submetido em: 06/09/2016
Instituição Proponente: FUNDACAO UNIVERSIDADE DE PERNAMBUCO
Situação da Versão do Projeto: Aprovado
Localização atual da Versão do Projeto: Pesquisador Responsável
Patrocinador Principal: Financiamento Próprio

Comprovante de Recepção: PB_COMPROVANTE_RECEPCAO_725909

— DOCUMENTOS DO PROJETO DE PESQUISA

- Versão Atual Aprovada (PO) - Versão 3
  - Pendência de Parecer (PO) - Versão 3
    - Documentos do Projeto
      - Comprovante de Recepção - Submissã
      - Cronograma - Submissão 4
      - Folha de Rosto - Submissão 4
      - Informações Básicas do Projeto - Subm
      - Outros - Submissão 4
      - Projeto Detalhado / Brochura Investigad
      - TCLE / Termos de Assentimento / Justif
    - Apreciação 4 - Universidade de Pernambuc
  - Projeto Completo

Tipo de Documento	Situação	Arquivo	Postagem	Ações

— LISTA DE APRECIAÇÕES DO PROJETO

Apreciação	Pesquisador Responsável	Versão	Submissão	Modificação	Situação	Exclusiva do Centro Coord.	Ações
PO	SILVIA REGINA SAMPAIO BEZERRA	3	06/09/2016	16/09/2016	Aprovado	Não	

— HISTÓRICO DE TRÂMITES

Apreciação	Data/Hora	Tipo Trâmite	Versão	Perfil	Origem	Destino	Informações
PO	16/09/2016 14:26:51	Parecer liberado	3	Coordenador	Universidade de Pernambuco/ PROPEGE/ UPE	PESQUISADOR	
PO	16/09/2016 14:25:35	Parecer do colegiado emitido	3	Coordenador	Universidade de Pernambuco/ PROPEGE/ UPE	Universidade de Pernambuco/ PROPEGE/ UPE	
PO	16/09/2016 14:25:06	Parecer do relator emitido	3	Coordenador	Universidade de Pernambuco/ PROPEGE/ UPE	Universidade de Pernambuco/ PROPEGE/ UPE	
PO	16/09/2016 14:24:13	Aceitação de Elaboração de Relatoria	3	Coordenador	Universidade de Pernambuco/ PROPEGE/ UPE	Universidade de Pernambuco/ PROPEGE/ UPE	
PO	15/09/2016 09:51:29	Confirmação de Indicação de Relatoria	3	Coordenador	Universidade de Pernambuco/ PROPEGE/ UPE	Universidade de Pernambuco/ PROPEGE/ UPE	
PO	08/09/2016 10:52:51	Indicação de Relatoria	3	Secretária	Universidade de Pernambuco/ PROPEGE/ UPE	Universidade de Pernambuco/ PROPEGE/ UPE	
PO	08/09/2016 10:52:25	Aceitação do PP	3	Secretária	Universidade de Pernambuco/ PROPEGE/ UPE	Universidade de Pernambuco/ PROPEGE/ UPE	
PO	06/09/2016 14:11:37	Submetido para avaliação do CEP	3	Pesquisador Principal	PESQUISADOR	Universidade de Pernambuco/ PROPEGE/ UPE	
PO	06/09/2016 09:41:26	Parecer liberado	2	Coordenador	Universidade de Pernambuco/ PROPEGE/ UPE	PESQUISADOR	Parecer homologado.
PO	06/09/2016 09:29:19	Parecer do colegiado emitido	2	Coordenador	Universidade de Pernambuco/ PROPEGE/ UPE	Universidade de Pernambuco/ PROPEGE/ UPE	

<< <   Ocorrência 1 a 10 de 26 registro(s)   > >>

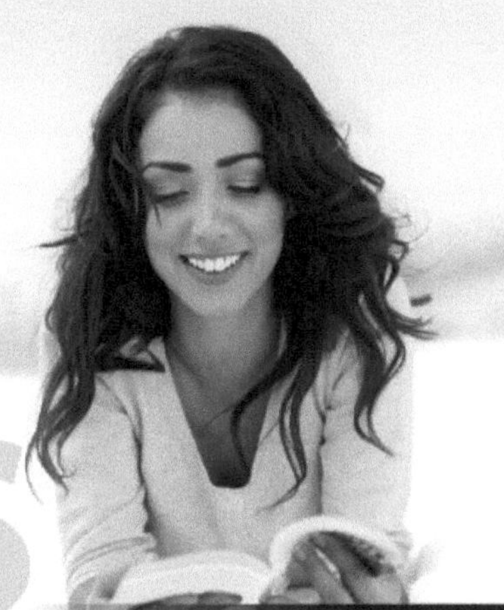

yes
I want morebooks!

Buy your books fast and straightforward online - at one of world's fastest growing online book stores! Environmentally sound due to Print-on-Demand technologies.

Buy your books online at
www.morebooks.shop

Kaufen Sie Ihre Bücher schnell und unkompliziert online – auf einer der am schnellsten wachsenden Buchhandelsplattformen weltweit! Dank Print-On-Demand umwelt- und ressourcenschonend produzi ert.

Bücher schneller online kaufen
www.morebooks.shop

info@omniscriptum.com
www.omniscriptum.com

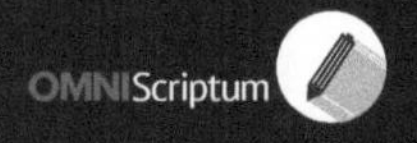

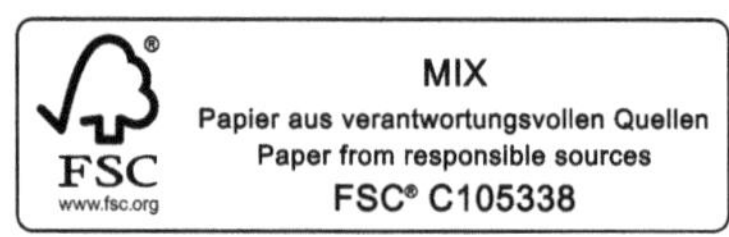

Printed by Books on Demand GmbH, Norderstedt / Germany